Patient Advocate's From Hell- by
L.J.Mora

Patient Advocates From Hell!

L.J.Mora

Patient Advocate's From Hell- by
L.J.Mora

Copyright©2016 L.J.Mora

All rights reserved

ISBN#13: 9781523487707

10: 1523487704

Patient Advocate's From Hell- by L.J.Mora

SYNOPSIS

I have worked in a Hospital for twenty-five years and have worked with some of the best Doctors and Nurses in New York.

I am not just saying that because I worked there. I am saying that because it is true.

My family got the bug to leave New York. That started a chain reaction of everyone else following them to the west coast- destination Las Vegas, Nevada.

I was the last one to relocate with my new husband.

I am sorry I did. Ever since I arrived here, Las Vegas has been taboo for me.

The healthcare here is no good! If you are thinking of going to a hospital here, transfer out to a different state!

Patient Advocate's From Hell- by L.J.Mora

In 2008, my cousin died, my mother died, my other cousin died and my husband died.

In 2009, my son shot himself.

In 2013, my father died.

This is where the story begins.

Patient Advocate's From Hell- by L.J.Mora

Author's Notes

Ever since I came here, I have noticed the difference in healthcare. They are so lax here it sickens me. I cannot stress this enough; if you are sick, please do not admit yourself to a local hospital here in Las Vegas. Please transfer out if you can.

When my husband was admitted into a local Hospital here, I met a woman I will call Emma.

She was going through the same thing as I was.

The respiratory therapist told her that her husband was dying.

That was only because she asked. I have written about this in my other books. My husband and son are in my book: Nightmare City-by L.J.Mora. The name definitely fits this town.

Patient Advocate's From Hell- by L.J.Mora

Table of Contents

Chapter 1-December 16, 2011 page-7

Chapter 2-January 03, 2012 page-9

Chapter 3-January 23, 2012 page-20

Chapter 4-January 25, 2012 page-22

Chapter 5-January 26, 2012 page-26

Chapter 6- January 27, 2012 page-29

Chapter 7- January28, 2012 page-33

Chapter 8- January 30, 2012 page-35

Chapter 9- February 02, 2012 page-38

Patient Advocate's From Hell- by L.J.Mora

Chapter 1

December 16, 2011

My father was admitted into Di Sierra Hospital here in Las Vegas for shortness of breath and chest pains. He was not getting good care at Di Sierra, because that is who they are, incompetent. However, incompetent became worse when they transferred him to Kindred Hospital.

Di Sierra tied his hands and feet up because they did not want to deal with him. In fact, they do not want to deal with anyone that is old.

Because that is just who they are- incompetent!

I looked for the Doctor and could not find him. They paged the Doctor and still, he did not answer.

Patient Advocate's From Hell- by L.J.Mora

Every time I was up there I could not find the Doctor!

The Asian Nurses could care less and blamed it on being busy.

My father was a good friend with one of the neighbors that lived across the street. I will call him Anthony.

I went up with Anthony to see my father and still, no Doctors could be found.

My father chased us away. He said, "I do not want you to see me like this- go away."

So, we backed off and left. That was a total waste of time, because when I inquired at the Nursing Station again, his Doctor was still not available!

I was beginning to think this was all a big game to them and a money making scheme. I know now, I am on the mark with this idea.

Patient Advocate's From Hell- by L.J.Mora

Chapter 2

January 03. 2012

Di Sierra Hospital transferred my father to Kindred Hospital Rehab. This Kindred Hospital is supposed to be for physical therapy. Today was my birthday and I was thinking of going out and treating myself to a birthday dinner. After all, it would be only me, eating by myself. I felt I deserved it after all the BS I have been through lately.

About 5:30 pm, I got a call on my cell phone.

It was a Doctor Diz from Kindred Hospital.

It figures, if I were looking for a Doctor, I would never find him, and now that I was looking to be alone, I find a damned Doctor!

I headed back to Kindred Hospital, where I just left. I spoke with this ditzy Doctor

Patient Advocate's From Hell- by L.J.Mora

Diz in the dining room. Not to eat, because I would do that after I left.

Doctor Ditzy Diz said, "I think you should be making plans for your father." I said, "Plans?"

Diz said, "Yes, I cannot help him."

I said, "May I remind you that Di Sierra Hospital admitted him here for extensive physical therapy."

Ditzy Diz said, "There is nothing I can do for your father. I think you should put him in a Group home."

"A group home? My father was admitted here for physical therapy what are you talking about?"
Ditzy Diz insisted I look into a Group Home. I did not even know what a Group Home was until I saw it myself.

My father was just admitted three hours ago and already they are trying to get rid of him.

Patient Advocate's From Hell- by L.J.Mora

At this point I was getting the bums rush.

The next day when I inquired about physical therapy the Nurses said he was getting 'bed exercises.'

I have never seen a physical therapist there with my father, ever.

They never got him up to walk.

When I visited my father, he was always sleeping. His hands and feet were always tied.

A week later, two female patient advocates approached me.

One was Kerry Wells and the other one was Irene Monk.

Ever since my father was admitted to this hell hole, Kerry and her sidekick that was always joined at her hip, Irene, were always trying to push these Group Homes on me.

Patient Advocate's From Hell- by L.J.Mora

I did not like the idea and wondered why the even sent him to Kindred. I did figure it out in the end, though.

I was approached by Taffy. A younger girl in her early twenties with an upbeat personality. She tried too hard.

She spoke with a little more tact, but I was not sold.

The next day, Taffy called me on my cell phone and convinced me to look at these Group Homes. Taffy said I had to look at the Group Homes because Kerry told her that.

I knew now, that both Kerry and Irene were manipulating Taffy.

My main concern now was why?

Why did they want to get rid of my father, so quickly?

I know the answer now, which I will reveal later on.

Patient Advocate's From Hell- by L.J.Mora

I called my aunt Terry and asked her to take me to look at these Group Homes.

I was picturing a huge Cottage like Nursing home with grassy grounds and Doctors and Nurses all over the place. An elegant dining room and even better Living room. Sort of like an Assisted Living Home.

Boy was I wrong!

I had two telephone numbers of the Nurses to two different Group Homes. My aunt and I were lost. We were riding around, blindly.

It was very dark on the street we rode down and we could not see the addresses. At this point, I felt a chill run down my spine. This street was spooky and I could not wait to get off it. My aunt suggested we look at the curb for the addresses.

That is usually where they are painted on.

Patient Advocate's From Hell- by L.J.Mora

I did not see anything that resembled a Nursing Home or an Assisted Care Home.

I did find the address and when I looked up, I immediately told her to 'drive on.' I told my aunt, "I am not even getting out. Just drive by!"

What we saw was a residence that belonged to a regular person, just like you and I. It was a house with a family. I pictured Asian cooking, every night. Children running around and noise from dogs barking.

As we were headed down the block, I got a call from the other Nurse.

I told her. "I am sorry. I cannot find the house." I hung up.

I did not know that the other Group home was on the same block!

Patient Advocate's From Hell- by L.J.Mora

I told my aunt, "forget about the second Group Home. I have seen enough! Let's just keep on going."

My cell phone rang again; it was the second Nurse calling me.

She said, "I can see you driving towards my house. A minute later, she practically jumped in the front of the car. We had no choice but to stop or run her over.

We chose to stop. I had no choice but to go through the motions.

My aunt waited in the car. I followed this Nurse up a bunch of rocks and walked into her house.

I saw a few elderly people in this house. There was a Christmas tree on the corner of the living room on my left. Straight ahead was the kitchen with a man cooking something. I could see him from the open divider. He said "hi," repeatedly. A woman was sitting on the couch in

Patient Advocate's From Hell- by L.J.Mora

another world. The Nurse then, showed me a Master bedroom, which was not a bad size. She told me the Master bedroom was being held for someone.

She then showed me a smaller room and said, "this will be your father's room."

I muttered, "the hell it will!"

My father also had Alzheimer's. The small room had a door that led into the street. I was afraid he would walk out of that door and into the street.

Where on earth do these people get their brains?

Not a good idea and NO common sense on their part!

I told this 'Nurse,' 'Thank you, but we have other places to see."

I could not wait to get out of there. I ran down those steps faster than the speed of lightening.

Patient Advocate's From Hell- by L.J.Mora

Taffy called me the next day. She said, "How did things go with the Group Homes?"

I said, "Do not ever do that to me again!"

Taffy said, "I am sorry, but Kerry and Irene made me do that." Taffy was mortified.

It was a shame that they dragged this young girl into all this Bull.

I started feeling bad for Taffy and said. "It is okay. It is not your fault. I will deal with Kerry and Irene!"

Every time Kerry and Irene called me, they put me on speakerphone and they were in the same office.

Then after I refused to put my father into their beautiful Group Homes that are run by CNA'S, not Nurses, that is when they both started showing their true colors.

Patient Advocate's From Hell- by L.J.Mora

Kerry called me the next day and said, "your father's coverage will not pay for the stay at Kindred Hospital.

I said, "My father has four different coverages. Would you like to take your pick?"

Kerry said. "His bill is going up every day! Tick-tock."

I said, "My father has Medicare, Humana Gold, Blue Cross/ Blue Shield and Ghi!"

Kerry said, "Well they do not cover the Kindred Hospital bill."

"Yes they do! I just called Medicare and Humana. Humana said that if my father owes anything at all, it would be only five dollars a day!"

This argument went on every damned day.

Kerry said, "You know, we charge over three thousand dollars a day. Tick- tock."

Patient Advocate's From Hell- by L.J.Mora

Every time she said Tick-tock, I wanted to punch her out! Kerry and Irene were two contemptable bitches!

They knew I was fighting this battle alone, but they never saw my aunt. They did not know I had a few family members left to defend me, if need be.

Patient Advocate's From Hell- by L.J.Mora

Chapter 3

January 23, 1012

Meanwhile, as all this BS was going on, I was looking into the Veterans Nursing home in Boulder City, Nevada. It is only 30 minutes away and it looked very nice in the pictures on the internet.

The Veterans Nursing home said they would accept my father, but he had to wait for a bed to become available.

I was okay with that and felt much better after my aunt and I saw the place.

I figured my father would be with people that were like him- Veterans! So he could feel like he had buddies, friends that were going through similar situations. Because most of them, did have Alzheimer's too.

The Veterans Nursing Home actually has a real dining room for the Veterans and for the families of Veterans.

Patient Advocate's From Hell- by L.J.Mora

They also had a dining room for the more serious Alzheimer's patients that needed a Nurse around while they ate dinner.

They had a huge Library and TV and a game room if they wanted to play board games or play card games.

They had a video room to watch movies.

They had a garden outside so you could soak up the sun.

There were two patients to a room and there were bathrooms and closets and draws in them.

They had a gift shop and also a small snack area where you could buy food from the counter and after hours, they had vending machines to buy snacks.

Now, it was just a matter of waiting for a room to become available.

Patient Advocate's From Hell- by L.J.Mora

Chapter 4

January 25, 2012

At 6:30 pm, I got a call from two of my favorite patient advocates.

You guessed it. Kerry and Irene! The two bitches from hell!

Kerry said, "Your father will have to be transferred to Red Rock!"

I said, "What is Red Rock besides a Casino?"

Kerry said, "Red Rock Rehab Center."

I said, "What? What the hell for?"

Irene chimed in, "we need to place your father ASAP!"

I said, "Why?"

Kerry went off in left field again and said, "his charges are going up. Now they are up to fourteen thousand dollars!"

Patient Advocate's From Hell- by L.J.Mora

Again, I said, "He has coverage they will pay for it!"

Kerry said, "no, they won't!"

I said, "yes, they will!"

At this point, I wanted to go through the phone and choke both of them!

I said, "why do you want to transfer him? You know he is going to the Veterans Nursing home, soon!

After fifteen minutes of badgering me, I finally got my answer, but I did not believe it.

Kerry said, "he needs to be weaned off of Ativan."

I said, "what? Are you kidding me?"

Kerry said, "he will be there for only five days.

Here is the address and phone number."

Patient Advocate's From Hell- by L.J.Mora

Again Kerry kept saying in a spooky tone of voice: "the charges for Kindred is three thousand dollars a daaaayyyy!"

Irene chimed in, as usual and said, "his charges are going up. Are you going to consent and send him to Red Rock Rehab?"

I said, "You know he is going to be transferred to the Veterans Nursing home. I do not want him to go anywhere else!"

Kerry said, "this will only be for five days."

I seriously think that they could say what they want, but once Red Rock had him, they (Kindred) would not take him back! I think that was their plan, all along. To pawn him off on someone else, even though they knew he was going to the Veteran's Nursing home.

I started thinking that if they got him hooked on a drug that he would have to be taken off it. So, I agreed to five days only!

After I agreed to the five days only, Irene said, "Now, I want you to tell Kerry what you just told me."

These two bitches were ruthless, but I did report them. They spoke to me as if I were a child.

I think these two were on drugs!

Chapter 5

January 26, 2012

I called Red Rock Rehab Center at 12pm. Here is how the scenario went down.

"Hello, Red Rock Rehab Center."

"Hello, I am looking for a patient. His name is Peter------"

"How do you spell the last name?"
I spelled my father's last name."

"I am sorry ma, am, but I have no one here by that name."

"Are you sure?"

"Yes, ma'am."
"Thank you." I hung up and felt better about that.

I called Kindred at 12:30 pm. I got Kerry's answering machine.

Patient Advocate's From Hell- by L.J.Mora

I called Kerry and Irene again at 1pm. I left message for them to call me back.

At 1:30 pm, I called Tam at the Veteran's Nursing home, in the Admissions dept.

Tam said, "I spoke to a Kerry at Kindred. She told me your father had to be weaned off Ativan."

I said, "Yes, she said he would be there for five days only."

Tam said, "I cannot take your father if he is hooked on drugs."

I said, "My father is not hooked on drugs."

Now, I was beginning to see what was going on here.

Both Kerry and Irene were making trouble for my father and me.

When Tam called Kerry back and asked her about it, Kerry said, "I never said that!"

Patient Advocate's From Hell- by L.J.Mora

Well, if Kerry 'never said that,' than why was she shouting at Tam?

I looked up Ativan online to see what it can do.

Chapter 6

January 27, 2012

"Ativan inj: To prevent withdrawal reactions, your Doctor may reduce your dose gradually. Report any withdrawal reactions immediately. Ativan Inj: is used to treat the following: induce temporary amnesia, anxious, repeated seizures with unconsciousness between episodes. Additional medication for calming."

When I read that, I already knew Kerry and Irene were lying!

My father never had any of those things wrong with him.

I called Kerry at 2pm. Still, no answer.

I called again at 2:10 pm, no answer.

At 2:30 pm, Kerry and Irene finally called me back.

Patient Advocate's From Hell- by L.J.Mora

I asked, "What is going on with my father?"

Kerry hesitantly said, "Red Rock did not accept your father."

She sounded mad and disappointed at the same time. I smiled because I knew I won half the battle, already.

Kerry then said, "If you do not place your father, we will keep tacking more charges on to your bill, daily."

I said, "They will pay for his bill."

Irene started shouting very unprofessionally, "No! They will not pay for his bill!"

At this point, both bitches were shouting at me over the phone.

Kerry said, "Are you going to call Medicare?"

I said, "I already did! Did he have any physical therapy while he was here? I don't think he did."

Patient Advocate's From Hell- by L.J.Mora

Both of them were mad because they knew I had their number. They knew I knew they were lying with their fabricated stories of BS!

Even though they knew he was an 86-year-old man with Alzheimer's, Kerry said, 'I do not know why you do not just take him home?"

I said, "I am not a healthcare professional to make that determination and besides, he has Alzheimer's!"

While I was arguing with these two bitches, I was still signing papers at the Veterans Nursing home to admit my father there.

I was happy my father was finally getting out of Kindred hellhole!

Before I got to the Veteran's Nursing Home, Ingrid called me up on my cell phone and said, "if you are such good buddies with Tam, why don't you tell her to pick up your father herself?"

Patient Advocate's From Hell- by L.J.Mora

Irene came out of left field with that one. I seriously think that both of them are possessed by the devil!

Shame on Doctor Diz for wanting to get rid of my father. I see that they are pushing their evil agenda on everyone. I wish more people would come forward and speak out against these evil asses that work at Kindred!

I will keep on posting online until I close them down! I will market the hell out of this book for all to read!

I will put this book in ALL LIBRARIES and warn others about the dangers of the elderly in these uncaring Hospitals!

I will even give out FREE copies!

Patient Advocate's From Hell- by L.J.Mora

Chapter 7

January 28. 2012

I went to see my father with my aunt. They had his hands and feet tied.

The wrist restraints were cutting off his circulation to his hands. It took me 10 minutes to get one wrist restraint off because of all the white tape that was fastened to them. I could not find a scissor or a CNA to help.

I did finally get them off.

Then, I noticed his food tray was on his table before we got there. They dropped his tray off and did not feed him. How did they expect him to eat with his hands tied?

They did not give him anything to eat or drink. Because he asked for a can of soda.

We did feed him while we were there. I asked the Nurse for a can of soda at about 6pm.

Patient Advocate's From Hell- by L.J.Mora

Someone muttered that they will be right in, but they never came into his room.

At 6:15, I asked another Nurse at the desk if my father could get a can of soda.

They said they would be right in.

They never came in!

At 6:30, I marched into the Nursing Supervisors office and told her what happened. She said she would be right there in his room in a few minutes.

No one ever came.

My aunt saw a CNA walk by and shouted: "how long do we have to wait for a can of soda?'

I would have gotten him a can of soda, but a Nurse at the Nursing station said it had to be thickened up before he drank it. Still, we had to wait.

He finally got his drink at 7pm!

Chapter 8

January 30. 2012

I knew my father was going to be admitted to the Veterans Nursing Home, so, I bought him two pairs of pajamas, two sets of underwear and two sets of t-shirts.

I made the mistake of placing them in his closet; because that is the first place, a thief would look to steal your belongings. I was on unemployment and could not afford much, but yes, someone did steal his new clothing.

No one knew where his clothing went. One CNA said that they transferred him to another room because housekeeping was doing the floors that night. In my opinion, what good is a clean place when you have incompetence running rampart? I looked in the room where he was originally and then, I looked in the room

Patient Advocate's From Hell- by L.J.Mora

where he was transferred again, just to make sure. I marched back into the Nursing Supervisor's office and reported it!

I said, "how can you transfer a patient without his belongings?"

The Nursing supervisor said that I would be reimbursed for the loss of his clothing.

I think I muttered something like; 'you mean for the stealing of his belongings.'

They did replace his clothes, but I liked the ones I bought better!

Again, we had another wild goose chase for thickened soda.

Well, if my father were okay enough to go home, according to Kerry, why are they giving him special meals like thickened soda and food that looks like colored flan?

Must be because he needs Nursing care? Hmmm, common sense!

Patient Advocate's From Hell- by L.J.Mora

They said he needs to eat that kind of food so he does not aspirate.

But, yet, Kerry wanted to know why I could not take him home! Go figure!

If he went home and ate and drank regular food, God knows what would have happened.

And no one could ever convince him, or anyone else for that matter, to eat their crap food!

Chapter 9

February 02. 2012

I arrived with my aunt at the Veterans Nursing home about five minutes to twelve.

A few minutes later, the ambulance brought my father in from Kindred.

He was in the hall on a gurney waiting for the drivers to sign off.

When he arrived there at the Veterans Nursing Home, he looked much older than he was. I noticed the black and blue marks were still on his hands and feet.

What we did not know was that there were more marks on his body.

When he got to his room, they treated him like a king. They walked him to the shower, washed his hair, and clipped his nails. In the process, the Nurses noticed that there were black and blue marks on his body and noticeable on his back.

Patient Advocate's From Hell- by L.J.Mora

When I walked into admissions, at the Veterans Nursing Home, I told them the problem I had with Kindred.

They told me that they too, were filing a complaint against Kindred. I asked for their phone number and told them, I am reporting Kindred, too!

I called up the hotline and sent the papers in to the address they gave me.

The Veteran's Nursing home said they did not like the way they received my father and thought there was foul play. My father needed long term care because of his Alzheimer's and Kindred was ready to let him go home because they "could not do anything for him." Doctor Diz's words!

Kindred never told me that my father's heart was working at 25 percent. The Veterans Nursing home were the ones that told me that.

Patient Advocate's From Hell- by L.J.Mora

A week later, I received a bill in my name for twenty-five thousand dollars!

It came from Kindred and was in a self-pay category!

And as for the Kindred Bill that Kerry and Irene put in my name for twenty- five thousand dollars, I called the Arizona Billing office and told the supervisor what happened with Kindred.

I told him that they hated my father and me and were trying to get rid of him from the very first day. I told the supervisor that Doc Diz said he 'could not help my father.' and I sent him all the info I am writing here in this book.

The supervisor of billing told me he would take care of the bill. That was after he heard and read my story.

After a week of my father being in the Veteran's Nursing home, he looked much better.

Patient Advocate's From Hell- by L.J.Mora

If you ever know of someone that is admitted into a Hospital here in Las Vegas, please do yourself a favor and keep a log of the daily things that happen. Take names, times, the Doctors they see. Write down what new Doctors they see and what they want to do. Write down everything! I hope you never have to use the info, but it would be good to have it in case you need it. Good Luck!

www.amazon.com/author/nylynlv

www.ingramcontent.com/pod-product-compliance
Lightning Source LLC
Chambersburg PA
CBHW020956180526
45163CB00006B/2386